21 Ways to Enjoy a Stress-Free Holiday Season

Praise for *21 Ways to Enjoy a Stress-Free Holiday Season*

"*21 Ways to Enjoy a Stress Free Holiday Season* is a very thorough outline of how to deal with holiday stress. Dr. Mommy shares real, honest to goodness tips that people can implement quickly and EASILY! This book is an amazing resource and everyone should have one."

—Kim Garst
SocialMediaBranding.com

"Finally a no-nonsense guide to getting through the holidays with less stress, more fun, and even some tips on saving money. Dr. Daisy is my go-to author and blogger for all things family and health-related and this book is no different. What I love most about it: *21 Ways to Enjoy a Stress-Free Holiday Season* is a short, quick read with do-able tips and essential reminders to take care of yourself while you're busy decking the halls and taking care of everybody else."

—Felicia J. Slattery, Author of *Cash in on Communication*

"Wow! This book is the greatest gift that you can give yourself. Not only are the tips great for having a stress free holiday, but some of them work well just for eliminating stress every day. Dr. Sutherland, I loved how you touched on everything that you could possibly think of that might add stress and gave so many creative ways to reduce it. I think this would make a great early Christmas present for others to buy for their extended family, I know I am! Not only will this help your readers, but just imagine how much more Amazing & stress free everybody's holiday would be if their families read it, too. Thanks, I am now ready to begin to prepare for the holidays with your book in hand and already feeling very relaxed!"

Susan Preston, Relationship Consultant
SusanCanHelpMe.com

"Dr. Mommy does it again! And just in time to help you actually enjoy the holidays. This little book is packed with a big punch in the form of 21 easily implementable strategies for decompressing, uncomplicating, and streamlining your holiday experience. The best part, is that the tips are life changes that you should implement year round, to maintain a more even pace to your life on a regular basis. A must-read for busy entrepreneurs, and super women wanna-be's."

Dr. Shannon Reece, The one trusted woman in a man's business world
www.DrShannonReece.com

"Just reading the titles of each of the *21 Ways to Enjoy a Stress-Free Holiday Season* will cause you to breathe sigh of relief. This is exactly the type of holiday season everyone wants and this book will help you get there—calm, refreshed, organized, and happy. What I enjoyed most was Dr. Sutherland's ability to provide workable solutions in a step-by-step format that is easy to follow and showed me how a stress-free holiday season is absolutely doable. You'll want to get several copies for gifts as I can't imagine you'll want to part with your own copy! Enjoy this book and enjoy your holidays!"

—Ann Vertel, Success Psychology Expert
AnnVertel.com

"Great Book! In *21 Ways to Enjoy a Stress-Free Holiday Season*, Dr. Mommy (Daisy Sutherland) shares tips that are often overlooked or not thought of. One key point is planning, and Dr. Sutherland gives outstanding instruction on how to plan efficiently and effectively. Why not make this year a stress-free holiday and pick up Dr. Sutherland's book today."

—Kelli Claypool, President & CEO of the Small Business and Learning Institute

21 WAYS

to enjoy a stress-free holiday season

Dr. Daisy Sutherland

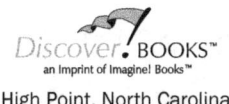

High Point, North Carolina

21 Ways™ Series, Book 3

Published by Discover! Books™
an Imprint of Imagine! Books™
PO Box 16268, High Point, NC 27261
contact@artsimagine.com

Imagine! Books™ is an enterprise of Imagine! Studios™
Visit us online at www.artsimagine.com

Copyright © 2011 Daisy Sutherland
Cover Design © 2011 Imagine! Studios™
Illustrations by Drawperfect, purchased at istockphoto.com

All rights reserved. No part of this publication may be reproduced or transmitted in any form or by any means, including informational storage and retrieval systems, without permission in writing from the copyright holder, except for brief quotations in a review.

ISBN 13: 978-1-937944-00-1
Library of Congress Control Number: 2011943611

First Discover! Books™ printing, November 2011

Dedication

For my husband and soul mate David,
who supports and loves me.

You are my true inspiration.

Acknowledgements

A special thank you to:

My family, who keep me motivated
and grounded, all at the same time.

My loving husband, David, for his
unstoppable support and love.

My dear friends, who believe in me and push
me until my head spins: Kristen Eckstein,
Felicia Slattery, and Kelli Claypool.

My heavenly father, who watches
over me, guides me, and shows
unconditional love to me.

Introduction

This book was written with you in mind. The stress I see people dealing with is often palpable, and my hope is that with the tips you find in this book, your life will become a little more calm and contented.

Stress is very real, and the holidays, which are meant to be a joyful time spent with family and friends, can often be among the most stressful times of your year. But with a little help, you can manage and ultimately reduce stress in your holidays and your life. The choice is yours to live a stress-free life and this little book will give you specific ways to achieve and *enjoy* a stress-free holiday.

Reclaiming your holidays is doable. You do not have to go around spinning in circles with no true direction. With a bit of pre-planning, you can reduce the effects of pressures that the many activities scheduled between Thanksgiving and the beginning of the year inevitably bring.

The first step in this journey is to remember that a great deal of the stress we feel at the holidays is of our own creation. Remember how exciting the holidays were when you were children? The thought of stress never entered your mind. Unfortunately, you can't turn back the clock to childhood, but you can implement some ways to lessen the stress and truly *enjoy* the holidays.

So stop, take a deep breath, and apply some of (or all of) the tips in this book. You will surely have a wonderful, stress-free holiday—as it was meant to be.

Happy Holidays!

Dr. Daisy Sutherland

WAY 1

Plan Ahead

Nothing is more stressful than having several activities scheduled all in one weekend, causing you to have to run from place to place without truly enjoying any event. The holidays are a wonderful time, but they can quickly become overwhelming if you neglect to plan ahead.

It's important to take out your calendar and place every little thing on it to avoid forgetting and losing your mind. And this applies to everyone in the family.

In an open area, keep a calendar designated as the "family calendar," where every family member can catalog individual holiday events. This system will also help with planning who's going where and when, as well as how they're getting there, and will help to avoid conflicts. The stress will come if you have failed to plan, so let's avoid that altogether by getting the family involved. Avoiding conflicts and overbooking is the goal, so planning ahead will help to lessen confusion as events begin to multiply.

Knowing ahead of time that a party is scheduled will also give you the opportunity to work extra hours if money is needed, giving you the opportunity to budget accordingly.

It's also important to remember that you don't have to attend every function, nor can you. Pick the ones that will be the least stressful and most enjoyable, perhaps ones with close friends or with people you don't get to see often enough throughout the year. Planning ahead allows you to pick and choose what activities to attend and which to decline, ultimately reducing your anxiety.

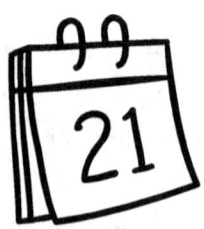

WAY 2

Essential Oils

There are times when you may need a little extra help to reduce your stress, and aromatherapy is a delightful and effective way to energize your mind and relax your spirit. Essential oils have been used for centuries and have wonderful healing effects.

Here are three wonderful essential oils you should not be without, especially during the holidays:

Lavender: This essential oil is known for its calming effects. It not only helps to balance and normalize body functions, but it also soothes and relaxes the mind. Lavender oil can be diffused into the air for a delightful aroma or applied directly on the skin. One way that we enjoy this oil in my household is to place a few drops in a spray bottle with distilled water. Take this solution and lightly mist your bed linens and you will fall into a deep sleep within minutes of laying your head on your pillow.

You may also find lotions and bath oils that contain lavender essential oil. Applying it directly to the skin or bathing in it will help to melt daily stressors away.

Peace and Calming: This oil is a blend of tangerine, orange, ylang-ylang, patchouli, and blue tansy. The aroma is gentle and fragrant, and when diffused in a room it will help calm tension and promote a sense of peace. This oil can be diffused into the air as well as applied directly to the skin. This is one that I carry in my purse for that added peace during stressful situations such as crowded stores or heavy traffic (perfect for use between November 1 and January 2). It's definitely one of my favorite stress-reducing essential oils.

Frankincense: This essential oil, used in religious ceremonies for thousands of years, has a sweet, warm, balsamic aroma. It helps to elevate the mind and reduce stress and despair. It can be diffused in the air for a delightful aroma, used topically, or ingested in a capsule form. In any of these forms, it will help to reduce your stress.

For more essential oils and to learn more about their benefits, visit DrMommyOnline.com/store

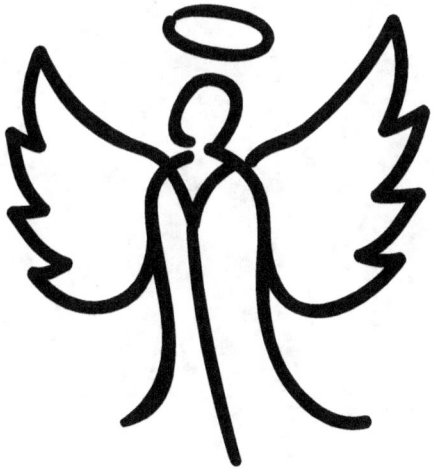

WAY 3

Ask for Help

One of the most important ways to reduce stress is to ask for help. This works not only during the holidays, but also all year round. Although many may think asking for help is a sign of weakness, it is actually a sign of courage.

If you don't have a close family member who can help, ask a neighbor, extended family member, co-worker, or church friend. There are always people willing to help you if you simply ask. Asking is often the most difficult and humbling part, but you may be surprised to find how many people are willing to help—and how willing you are to help in return.

Some tasks where help is always needed:

Decorating the house

Many will go all-out decorating the entire house both inside and out, so instead of going crazy doing it yourself, ask for help. You can even make a party of it, which relieves stress and brings back some of the childlike joy of the holidays.

Cleaning the house

Once your house is decorated, the cleaning part comes into play. Actually, it always comes into play. Don't stress over keeping your home spotless. Instead, enlist your family members in helping to keep things tidy. You may also opt to hire a cleaning service once a month or just during the holiday season to clean up after a party or after your major decorating is finished.

Wrapping gifts

Save yourself a lot of time and stress and have your gifts wrapped at the store where you purchase them. Many stores offer free gift-wrapping services, or nonprofits often offer for-donation services at a table by the registers.

If gift wrapping is not offered, ask others to help wrap gifts, or, better yet, use gift bags. See Way 16 for more wrapping tips.

Baking

Whether you are baking cookies or cakes, or cooking entire meals, asking for help will reduce your stress. You can ask for help with the baking itself, the cleanup, or reading of the recipes to make your measuring go faster. Whatever the task, get others involved and make a family affair out of it. And being with others instead of remaining isolated in the kitchen can be a real help.

Shopping

During the holiday season, the stores will be overly crowded, which can cause your stress levels to increase. Ask a friend to accompany you on your trip. Make a day of it and have a special lunch. You'll be surprised how much you will accomplish with little to no stress, and it could even be fun!

Childcare

Shopping with children can be *extremely* stressful. Hire a babysitter to watch the children while you shop. The children will be safe and entertained at home and you will have peace of mind while shopping. You can also shop free of worries that they will see their gifts and spoil your holiday surprise.

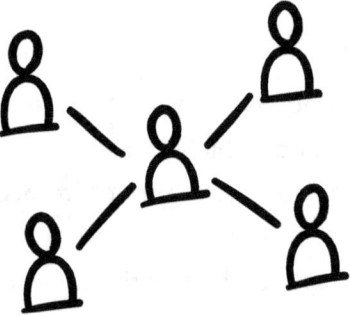

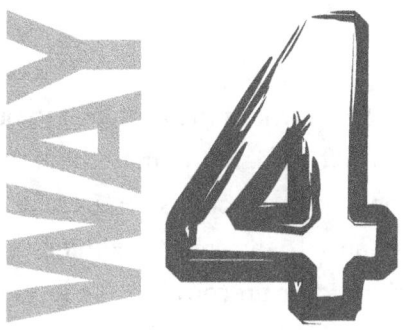

Shop Early

If you're like most people, shopping is the most stressful part of the holidays. However, you can reduce this stress by shopping early. Of course we all have good intentions and plan to shop early, but for some reason it rarely works. Here are some tips that may help:

Start shopping early

Sounds crazy, but many items such as decorations and ornaments will go on sale even before the end of the year. Take that opportunity to stock up early. You can take advantage of some wonderful discounts.

Gift cards

For the person who is the toughest to purchase for, get a gift card. Some may think these are impersonal, but recipients are usually grateful for the chance to pick out something they want but perhaps didn't receive. The variety available is incredible—from home improvement shops to movie tickets. And get them early, so that you can check this off your list.

Here's a tip shared by a friend: Every time you go grocery shopping, pick up a gift card. By the end of the year you will have a variety of gift cards to choose from for birthdays, anniversaries, and, of course, the holidays.

Purchase holiday cards early

Many holiday cards are available as early as September. Start addressing them early and they'll be ready to send without any stress. Set yourself a goal of addressing a few each week so that you aren't overwhelmed.

Shop online

Avoid the crowds and long lines and shop online. Sometimes items bought online will come wrapped and ready to give, and often deals for free shipping are advertised during the holiday season.

Visit discount and warehouse stores

Many of these stores will sell items in bulk at a discounted price, which is easier on you and your budget.

Order your ham or baked goods

If you have a party to attend and simply don't have time to bake, take advantage of the shops that offer to cook for you. Order your baked ham or cookies early, place the pickup date on your calendar, and you're good to go.

Cyber Monday

Shop from the comfort of your own home in your pajamas and avoid dealing with the crowds the day after Thanksgiving. Many big retailers will have sales on the Monday following Thanksgiving. Shopping at home is more comfortable and convenient and will certainly reduce your stress.

Clearance

Why pay the retail price when you can find incredible buys in the clearance rack? Stock up on decorations and candles, as well as items that never go out of style, and store them for use next year.

You'll notice that implementing some, if not all, of these tips will help to reduce the stress that accompanies shopping. Having a plan before tackling the stores is always wise, not to mention cost effective.

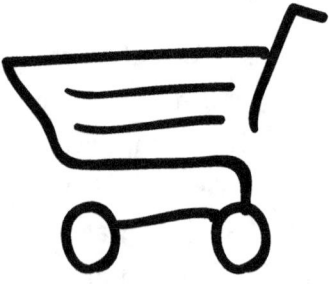

WAY 5

Less Is More

Who says you have to have more decorations outside your home than anyone else in your neighborhood? Do you really want to pay the huge electric bill that comes along with it? How about the time it takes to pull out all the decorations in the first place, not to mention taking them down after the holidays? Here are some tips for stress-free decorating:

Books

Consider decorating with books that have a seasonal touch. Display an illustrated volume of *A Christmas Carol* on your living room coffee table or fireplace mantel. A basket full of children's holiday books with a pretty festive bow makes a great decoration piece as well.

Go monochromatic

Choose a color such as red, blue, or green and run with it. Take an empty vase and fill it with red ornaments of all shapes and sizes and you have a wonderful centerpiece. Choose white lights to wrap around your banister and frame your mantel for a beautiful, clean look.

Use what's on hand

Create a gallery of pretty packages by wrapping existing frames with festive foil gift wrap. Place the frames back on their original hooks and you have a creative and festive gallery.

Fabrics

Even if you don't sew, fabrics come in handy for decorating. Choose a festive fabric for a table covering or to use as a tree skirt. After use it can simply be washed and stored for the next year.

Use natural elements

Grab some pinecones or pine tree branches to display on your mantel or in a bowl. This Old World–style decoration is wonderfully natural and will make your house smell divine.

Take your time

Remember that decorating does not have to be completed all in one day. Pace yourself and take your time. Seeing your home transformed in stages will make it all worth it.

Small is better

Many times we think that the largest tree is the best, but don't underestimate smaller versions. Miniature potted evergreens add a lovely touch to the fireplace area or a hallway. After the holidays, plant them outside.

It's amazing what changing your mindset and implementing smaller-size decorating themes will do to reduce your stress. Holidays are meant to be enjoyed with family and friends, and becoming anxious about a massive decorating scheme steals that joy. Plus, with small-scale plans you won't have to bribe anyone to hang millions of ornamental lights on your home for a mere three weeks.

WAY 6

Treat Yourself

It's important to remember that, although the hustle and bustle of the holidays are upon you, your daily routine should not end. Your everyday practices help to calm and center you, and you will still need them to get through this busy season.

If that doesn't work, then you must—and I repeat, you *must*—schedule downtime for yourself. If you have to go as far as placing it on your calendar, then do it! During this downtime be sure to:

Get a massage

Oh my, a massage will work wonders for your entire body and mind! Holiday stress will tense up your muscles and a massage will do the trick to relax your body and mind to be completely refreshed.

Date your mate

If you are stressed, you can bet your mate is as well. Make sure to spend some quality time with him or her, whether for lunch or dinner, and talk about anything other than shopping, decorating, or holiday parties.

Go to the movies

Get away from the rush of the season and enjoy a movie. Don't just rent a movie; actually go the theatre. Getting out of the house will help you relax and focus on having fun amidst home-based activities that tend to be stressful, especially if you have greeting cards to address and presents to wrap.

Read

If you enjoy reading before bedtime, then continue to do so and don't put it off in favor of another holiday chore. Reading will help you escape from the stress and allow you to get lost in someone else's story.

Take a bath

Nothing is more relaxing than a warm bath—a bubble bath or one with fragrant essential oils (see Way 2). You will soak away your tension and truly forget about the holiday stressors you—and everyone else—may be experiencing.

Mani-pedi time

Remember to treat yourself to a manicure and/or pedicure. You shouldn't neglect yourself and this is a perfect way to relax and reduce your stress.

Go for a walk

Nothing will relax the mind more than simply going for walk in the neighborhood or park. Going outdoors will refresh your mind and spirit and get you back into the holiday mood.

Treating yourself is something you should schedule into your normal monthly routine. Your health and wellness will be maintained when you take time to unwind and simply do what you enjoy. Remember, it doesn't have to break the bank, but it should bring a sense of peace and calming.

WAY 7

The "B" Word

The famous "B" word—budgeting. During this season be sure to set a budget ahead of time and, most importantly, stick to it. Nothing is more stressful than receiving the credit card bills in January and then taking an entire twelve months, or more, to pay them off.

Budgeting doesn't mean you have to go on the "cheap." Instead, implement a few tips and tricks to keep your holiday season stress free and budget friendly. The goal to enjoying the holidays is to eliminate stress, and employing some of these tips will surely help:

Make a list

It won't be difficult to stay within your budget if you make a list first. List those you want to purchase gifts for and determine an amount you are willing to spend, and then stick to your list.

Avoid eating out

As much as you'd like to go out and celebrate each weekend, it will begin to add up. Instead, purchase special ingredients and make meals at home. Experiment by mimicking some of your favorite restaurant meals for a fraction of the cost.

Be creative with your gifts

Consider giving distant relatives photos in a frame instead of purchasing items they may or may not use or need. Hobby Lobby runs continuous sales on their photo frames at 50 percent off. Digital photo frames are also great because you can add more than one photo. A calendar with photos of your children each month is another great gift idea you can create at just about any photo printing shop.

Give the gift of time

One of the best gifts you can give a family member or child is special time with you. Make up certificates for that special someone for "a special date night" or "a trip to the movies together." Nothing is more meaningful than quality time, and that will always fit in your budget.

Budget your time

Although you may think you have all the time in the world, life always seems to get in the way. Keep track of your time and monitor how long particular tasks take. Proactive time management will help you keep your sanity.

Budgeting doesn't have to be a bad word or leave a bad taste in your mouth. In fact, when you get into the practice of determining your budget and sticking to it, you will notice something truly magical—less stress and more money in the bank.

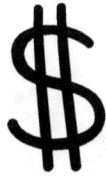

WAY 8

Serve Others

During this season, and every season, there are many people in need. The holidays tend to accentuate that need because of the spending sprees some go on at this time of year. A great way to reduce the stresses you may be feeling is to help and serve others. Consider having your family and friends join you on this venture and making it a tradition. Here are a few ways to serve others this holiday season:

Visit shut-ins

There are many who may not have the ability to go out, much less go shopping. These people are usually elderly. Visit a nursing home or assisted living facility and bring along others to read to them and sing carols. It will lift their spirits and give you a sense of satisfaction.

Children's homes

There are many children in your own community who are without a family of their own, and this is a wonderful time of year to visit these children and bring gifts. Call the facility first and ask for a list of items that they need. Together with your children or youth group, gather needed items and bring them to these wonderful children. When you see their eyes light up, you will recognize the true meaning of this season.

Hospitals

Call your local hospitals and get involved by donating gifts, food items, or time. In addition to the patients, think of the nurses and doctors who are not able to leave and spend time with their families. This is a perfect opportunity for you to serve them.

Meals on Wheels

This great organization delivers food to the elderly and offers a great way for you to serve.

They are always looking for volunteers to cook, gather food items, prepare the baskets, and deliver meals. The recipients look forward to the visits and the goodies, and it's another wonderful way to forget about your stress and serve others.

Donate to those less fortunate

Many families don't have enough money to purchase gifts for their children or prepare a holiday meal. Consider ordering an extra turkey or ham and putting together a holiday basket for a family in need. There are many organizations that have lists of families whom you can serve. Contact the local Salvation Army or Goodwill, or local churches, for more information.

Choose one of the above activities to add to your holiday tradition this year and watch your stress melt away as your focus shifts to others.

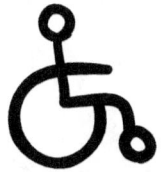

WAY 9

Use the Magic Word

The magic word I'm referring to is "No." During this holiday season you will without a doubt be approached to participate in something, help someone, or donate of your time to your church, school, family—the list goes on. If you have a problem using this magic word, then you will experience the inevitable—stress.

It's important to know your commitments and keep track of them. Do this by placing them on your calendar or electronic device. You can then easily check your schedule and honestly tell those requesting your help that you are not available.

This magic word will not only reduce your stress, but it will also allow you to truly relax. If you are one of those individuals that everyone comes to for help because you can't use this magic word, consider using the following phrase that has always worked for me. Next time you are cornered by the PTA president of your child's school or a co-worker to do yet another project, instead of hesitating and giving in to their requests, say this phrase instead: "That sounds wonderful, but I can't say 'yes' to that at this time."

Since the word "no" seems to have a negative connotation, using the reverse such as in the saying above will catch the other person by surprise. It's important to say this phrase with a smile and you"ll be surprised when the person asking for your time will not ask why or try to coax you but will accept your answer.

Reduce your stress by using this magic word more often and, if you have difficulty using it, try the "can't say yes" phrase. Always remember, saying "no" to some things will leave the door open to say "yes" to things that matter the most. See Way 8 for a few things to say "yes" to that will help reduce your holiday stress.

WAY 10

Capture the Memories

During this time of year it seems that everyone is rushing to get professional photos of their families taken. Do you know how stressful that can be? Standing in line for hours with grumpy children all dressed up? Here are some great ways to avoid this needless stress:

Schedule in advance

You will miss the rush of people who wait until the last minute to have photos taken if you schedule your photo earlier in the year. Decide what theme or outfits you will all wear in advance and schedule your appointment for

September. You'll be glad you did. While everyone else is rushing around with back-to-school events, you will be one step ahead with your holiday photos complete.

Hire a college student

There are many photography majors who need to fill their portfolios. Not only will they be reasonably inexpensive, but they also can come to your home or take outdoor photographs.

Be creative

Who says you need to do still shots? Consider creating videos of your family and sending them to family members who live in other states. In this age of technology, you don't have to always settle for the same old thing.

Take photos yourself

Yes, you read that correctly. Take the photos yourself by using the timer device on your camera. If you don't have a tripod, you can place the camera on a shelf, cabinet, or even a pile of boxes or books and have fun! Be sure to save some of the bloopers, as everyone loves to see those and laugh at one another.

The most important part of this entire process is to have fun. Finding creative and unique ways to capture memories will increase your joy and reduce your stress. You can also get your children, family, or friends involved, a relief for you and a treat for them.

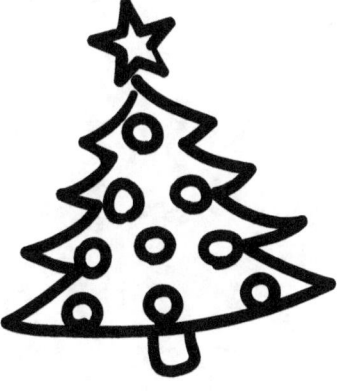

WAY 11

Outward Bound

Traveling can be stressful any time of the year, and it tends to be even more so during the holidays. However, by setting some plans in place you may avoid the headaches and stress altogether. Here are some tips to make your holiday travels more enjoyable for all:

Make a list

This little tip has helped me on many occasions when packing for a large family. Make a list of every item that you need to pack, down to the toothbrush and hair dryer. You'll be surprised the little things you will forget if you don't place them on your list. This list will not only ensure you pack every item needed, but it will save you time as well. You can also save a "master list" on your computer and print it off every time you take a trip.

Pack smart

Aside from your luggage, pack a separate bag with toothbrushes and everyone's sleepwear. The first night when you arrive at your destination, this one bag with all the essentials is much easier to handle than going through each individual suitcase.

Stay safe

If you're traveling by vehicle, make sure your vehicle is in good running order—tires all filled, oil changed, and fluid levels all checked. Being prepared will help to reduce stress levels. Another important tip is to check your local auto club with regard to road conditions. Also have a map handy. Don't simply rely on your GPS.

Avoid airport hassles

Simplify your traveling by arriving at the airport up to two hours early for domestic flights and up to three hours for international flights.

Instead of leaving your car in overnight parking, ask a friend or relative to drive you to the airport.

Travel-proof gifts

With all the security restrictions at the airports, avoid any needless stress by purchasing gift cards or gift certificates. If that won't do, consider having the gifts mailed to your destination so they are waiting there when you arrive. Shipping gifts will also leave more room in your suitcase.

Traveling doesn't have to become a nightmare. Instead, implementing these tips will help you look forward to traveling and take time to enjoy every minute.

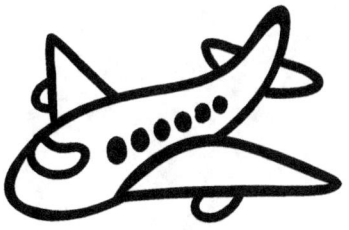

WAY 12

Time to Play

Make time to go outside and release all the energy that tends to get pent up, energy that leads to stress. When you are active, it boosts your energy and your mood, so don't slow down just because the holiday routine may be a little different.

If at all possible, it's important to not change your routine. Continue to take your daily walks or your visits to the health club. If you have children, make sure to go outside and enjoy the crisp weather with them.

Is it snowing? Go outside and build a snowman, go sledding, or make snow angels. Make the time to go outside or simply take a break from the craziness that surrounds the holiday season.

If the weather doesn't allow you to go outside, have fun inside. Take out some of the old board games, blow off the dust, and play. How about the fun game of Twister? Not only will you be challenging yourself by twisting in awkward positions, but your family will have fun, too!

Let your inner child come out. How about Legos? You'll be amazed at how relaxing playing and creating with Lego pieces can be. Or simply color or build puzzles—these activities can be quite soothing.

Play some holiday music, make some hot chocolate, and enjoy your family. Too often the many activities of the holidays lead to your running around and forgetting the people that matter the most. Make sure to set some special time aside for them and you to simply have fun!

The possibilities are endless—you just need to stop, breathe, and enjoy!

WAY 13

They Have It All

Do you have people on your list who seem to have it all? Those people are certainly the hardest to purchase for, and thinking about it leads to stress. Consider some of the following ideas for people who have it all or claim they don't want a gift:

Gift cards

Although they may seem impersonal, gift cards can be very handy. It's best to either get one to their favorite shop or a generic one like a VISA gift card that can be used wherever they please. See Way 4 for another great gift card tip.

Item of the month club

There are many of these types of memberships available, such as book of the month, candle of the month, beer or wine of the month, cheese of the month, flower of the month, and the list goes on. Determine what this person enjoys and surprise him or her with this unique gift.

Customized book

If this person is an avid reader, consider this unique gift. At Custom Classics (CustomizedClassics.com), you can create a special edition of a classic book and have this person become one of the main characters.

Personalize it

Although they may have everything, they may not have it personalized. The possibilities are endless, including robes, jewelry boxes, coffee mugs, or luggage.

Donate your services

Everyone loves free services. Consider creating certificates that offer this person free babysitting services, house cleaning, errands for the day, or a home-cooked meal.

Whatever you decide, don't allow this person to stress you out over a gift. Be creative, use your imagination, and surprise him or her. After all, it is the season of giving, and the best gifts come from your heart and creativity.

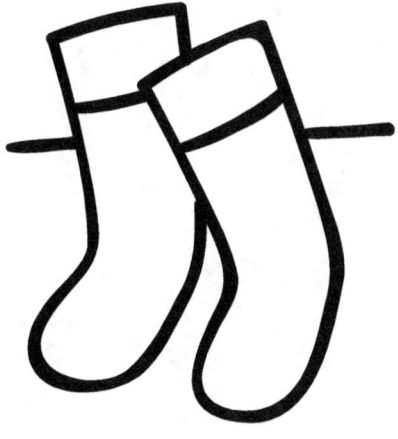

WAY 14

Pass the Torch

If you find yourself baking or wrapping gifts at midnight, it's time to lower your expectations and pass the torch.

Make a list

No one said that *you* must do it all. So make a list and have your partner or significant other do some of the shopping.

Give the kids scissors

Have your children help with the wrapping. Yes, the children! Remember, it doesn't have to be perfect and this is a great bonding time. See Way 16 for more ideas on how to delegate wrapping.

Crafting

Get some fun craft items and have the children create crafts for the holidays as well as gift cards and labels. Let them shine and show their creativity.

Pass on Santa

Let someone else play Santa and allow others around you to join in on the fun. Allow them to organize the gifts under the tree, and on Christmas morning let them hand out the gifts.

Let them cook

Teach your children all the traditional cookies, pies, and meals you've made for years and let them help you. Once they have mastered your tips and recipes, it's time to pass the torch and let them take over some of these traditions.

Passing the torch on items you've done for years will allow you some extra time to devote to special activities you'd like to participate in. Perhaps you just want to relax and enjoy some hot chocolate by the fire. This will all be possible if you pass the torch and let go.

Learn to let go of perfectionism and allow others to help. You'll find that you can have a more peaceful and enjoyable holiday by sharing it. See Way 3 for more ideas on how to ask for help.

WAY 15

Surviving the Social Whirl

In order to curb your stress level, try to keep your social gatherings small and intimate. Get together with a few of your closest friends or relatives for the holidays. Choose to attend large get-togethers or parties at another time of the year, when you and your guests will have fewer commitments and will actually enjoy the event.

Take advantage of the timesavers

Order your favorite pie from your local bakery or sandwich platter from your favorite deli. Ordering some of the extras such as appetizers, breads, and desserts will make your preparation

WAY 16

De-stress Wrapping

Some of the most time-consuming and stressful moments of the entire holiday season are spent wrapping gifts. Once you've completed your purchase list, the wrapping comes into play. Don't do it alone!

Start wrapping early

Don't wait until the last minute to wrap. Once you purchase an item wrap and label it; and save the ribbons and bows until the end.

Find free wrapping

Ask the department store clerk about free gift wrapping. Many won't advertise this service, so be sure to ask.

Use gift bags

Whenever possible, use gift bags. These come in very handy for odd-shaped gifts and those that are too large or too small to wrap.

Use kid art

Have the children decorate craft paper with their unique drawings, stickers, and stamps, then use that paper to wrap gifts.

Put teens to work

Enlist teens' help with the wrapping. They are younger and have more energy, so be wise and allow them to help.

Find a charity

Seek out charity gift-wrapping services. Many nonprofit organizations will set up booths at malls or craft shows and wrap presents for a fee. Take advantage of their services and you'll save yourself one major task while contributing to a worthy cause.

Stock up

Take advantage of all the sales and stock up on wrapping paper, tape, and gift bags at the end of the season. Nothing is more frustrating than running out of supplies with the job half finished. Also save bags and bows from previous years to recycle the next year.

Whatever you do, don't sit on the floor to wrap gifts. It may seem like a great idea at first because of all the room to spread out, but your back and legs will suffer and that will make it difficult for you to enjoy the holidays. Instead, use a table to wrap items and avoid the floor!

Have fun! Play festive music or your favorite DVD while you wrap gifts. Be sure to treat yourself and those helping you with delicious hot chocolate topped with whipped cream to stay energized.

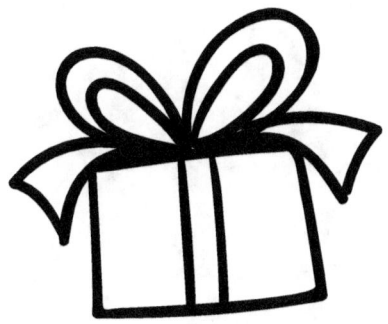

WAY 17

Do It Together

The holiday season is always more enjoyable when you can share it with others. Instead of taking on all the tasks yourself, let others help you.

If you are in charge of coordinating a holiday party at work, school, or the neighborhood, or if you are responsible for planning a family event, be sure to have plenty of people to help you. Not only will it run more smoothly, but you will also be less overwhelmed in the end.

Make sure to have a list of all the materials needed, such as decorations, a tree, lights, food, and music. Assign the different people on your team their own tasks and set them free. This means don't micromanage and hover over them while they decorate the tree or set out the cookies. They may do it differently than you would, but they will own it and enjoy it, and you will free yourself from the burden of doing it all.

No one wants to remember being the only one doing the work and being miserable instead of joyous, so focus on trying to have fun doing it all together. Not only will it create memories, but it will also make your life easier. In fact, it can turn into a tradition.

Having everyone participate makes an event memorable. If you don't have any traditions as of yet, there's no better time than now to start a new one that doesn't include you carrying the biggest load of work.

Recruit your family and friends to decorate together, cook together, and merely enjoy one another's company. People naturally want to help, but they won't want to step on your toes. So this season, let go, allow others to help, and watch your stress melt away. Doing it together will make you look forward to the holidays instead of dreading them.

WAY 18

Watch the Sweet Tooth

The holiday season brings on many parties and celebrations. With those celebrations you will find many delicious treats that will tempt you to indulge. If you succumb to your weakness, you will find yourself ill from overeating and stress will begin to build up.

Instead of overindulging on the many treats available, pace yourself. No one says you must not enjoy the treats. However, enjoying treats in moderation will be much more enjoyable in the end.

Don't wait until the beginning of the year as to start a New Year's resolution. You can enjoy your holidays just fine, including all the treats of the season, by exercising just a bit of self control. No one knows your body better than you. So, if you know that you will feel sick after three cookies, then control yourself and stop at two. If you're invited to a party that you know will have many sweets, consider eating a healthy meal first so you are not as tempted to overindulge.

Drinking water will also help you to curb the temptation to eat too many sweets. It will give you the satiated feeling so you will limit your intake. You can do it!

If you do find yourself hovering over the dessert table, make sure to stay active. Dance off the added calories and have fun! Again, you know what it will take to make you happy. Focus on that and your stress levels will be reduced.

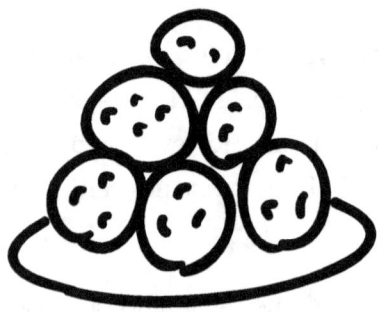

WAY 19

Keep the Rituals

As silly as it may sound, it's important to keep family rituals intact during the holiday season.

Thanksgiving

If your family enjoys going around the table giving thanks, then continue to do so. Whatever your ritual is for this special day, don't allow the stress of the holidays to interfere with your family traditions. Continue to build memories and take the time to enjoy the day completely. The dishes will wait while you sit down to a game of football or watch a favorite holiday movie.

Decorating the tree

Keep the tradition of decorating the tree alive or create a new one starting this year. Put on some tunes and decorate the tree together with your family, or invite friends over to trim the tree. If it's a large tree, you may want to decorate in stages. If you have precious collectible ornaments, consider having a separate tree for the children to decorate. Another idea is to have a miniature tree in each room that your children can decorate. The possibilities are endless!

Singing carols

Keep singing carols around the neighborhood. But don't limit it to the neighborhood; go to friends' homes and get them excited for the season. Or consider visiting a nursing home. You may brighten someone's evening and make a positive impact on a life.

Read the Christmas story

Truly make this an event, one that you stop and create time for. Prepare some hot cocoa and gather around for a reading of this story. Have each family member participate to create some new traditions. You can also record yourself or a loved one reading this story, so these precious voices will be remembered reading it in years to come.

Bake together

Create some long-lasting memories by baking together. If not baking, how about decorating a gingerbread house? The children will be able to share their creativity and you'll be able to take a break from the rushing this holiday season tends to bring.

Watch a holiday movie

There are many holiday favorites that will bring the family together. Some of our favorites are *A Charlie Brown Christmas*, *Rudolph the Red-Nosed Reindeer*, and *Elf*. Choose some of your favorites, and enjoy with some popcorn and warm apple cider.

Go see the lights

One of our all-time favorite family traditions is to visit the surrounding neighborhoods and admire their light displays. Some folks go way out, but you don't have to. Take in the sights and enjoy some delicious candy canes while you visit and admire.

WAY 20

Postpone Festivities

No, don't postpone the holidays altogether, but there are so many parties that take place during the month of December that you can't possibly attend all of them. If you attempt to make everyone happy, you will end up more stressed than when you started. Instead of trying to squeeze in one more party, consider planning one for the New Year.

There isn't a written rule that parties must occur before January 1. While everyone is stressing over the many parties to attend, consider scheduling yours for an evening in mid-January. Once the rush has calmed down and the family and friends have returned from their trips, a toned-down party will surely be welcome. Here are some post-holiday party ideas:

Plan a potluck dinner

This is a perfect gathering for co-workers or friends who were too busy to get together in December. The bonus is that this gathering will truly be about the people: no gifts necessary and no added stress of decorations.

White elephant party

These parties are always fun and interactive. This is also a great way to get rid of the odd gifts or duplicates you may have received. Each guest will bring a gift they are willing to trade for someone else's gift and the fun begins. Do an Internet search for some white elephant gift exchange activity ideas.

Un-decorating party

Gather a few friends for a light dinner and recruit their help in un-decorating the tree. This is a fun time to simply relax with friends after a busy holiday season.

Organize a group outing

If you don't want to deal with hosting yet another party, organize a concert or movie outing with special friends, with cocktails at your home afterward.

The holidays may be over, but you can still celebrate a new year in the company of family and friends.

WAY 21

Reason for the Season

With all the craziness the holidays tend to bring, let's not forget the reason for this season. Not only is it a time to give thanks, but it should also be a time to simply enjoy your family and friends. No one wants to spend time with someone who is completely stressed and can't simply sit down for a few seconds.

This is a time to relax and reflect on the entire year. Perhaps there are things you would have done differently, but don't dwell too long on those. Instead, focus on the goodness that the year brought you. Look at how big your children have grown and the many friendships you made.

Look at how much *you* have grown from the beginning to the end of the year. We all have life lessons that we learn from each year (for more *Life Lessons* see my book of that same title). Focus on the goodness and simply have fun!

Is there something you could have done differently? Is there a way you can implement that for the coming year? Who says you have to wait for the New Year? You can start today making a difference not only in your life, but also in the lives of others.

Christmas is also special to me and to millions of other people around the world because it commemorates the birth of Jesus Christ—the greatest gift of all!

Remember that this is supposed to be the season of love, joy, and peace—not stress and anxiety. Make some time to read the Christmas story and reflect on what Christmas means to you. And if your thoughts and expectations about Christmas and gift giving aren't what you'd like them to be, do what you can to change them for next year!

Conclusion

Whew! Do you feel better? My hope is that the tips shared in this book will help you truly enjoy the holiday season.

It's natural to feel a bit overwhelmed, but it's important to find ways to reduce the stress before it completely takes over. Most importantly, enjoy this beautiful season, forget the past, focus on today, and plan for the year ahead.

Implement some of the tips shared in this book and make sure to make time for *you*. Pampering yourself is very important to your overall health and well-being and definitely a way to reduce your stress!

Enjoy this holiday season!

Merry Christmas and Happy New Year!

Resources

Order Essential Oils:
DrMommyOnline.com/store

High quality, inexpensive photo frames:
HobbyLobby.com

Meals on Wheels
MOWAA.org

Customized Books:
CustomizedClassics.com

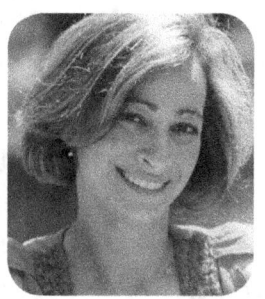

About the Author

Dr. Daisy Sutherland is the Founder and CEO of *Dr. Mommy Online*. Her main mission and goal is to IME—*Inspire, Motivate & Encourage*—you to be the best you can be in health, wealth, and sanity!

She is a Doctor of Chiropractic, author, speaker, and radio personality, but most importantly she is a devoted wife and mom to five. She understands the trials of life and has overcome many, and because of this she is determined to help others through this wonderful journey we all call life!

She encourages you to not dwell on the past and allow it to form who you are today. Instead, you should learn from past so that you can become the greatness you were created to be. This is her motto and through her writings, audios, and speaking engagements, she continues her mission of inspiring, motivating, and encouraging others.

For more of what Dr. Mommy has to offer visit her site: DrMommyOnline.com

Do you feel lost?

Are you simply dragging through your week?

Do you have difficulty finishing projects?

Are the kids wearing you out?

Get FREE instant access to Dr. Daisy's report

7 Simple Ways to Get Motivated

DrMommyOnline.com/motivated

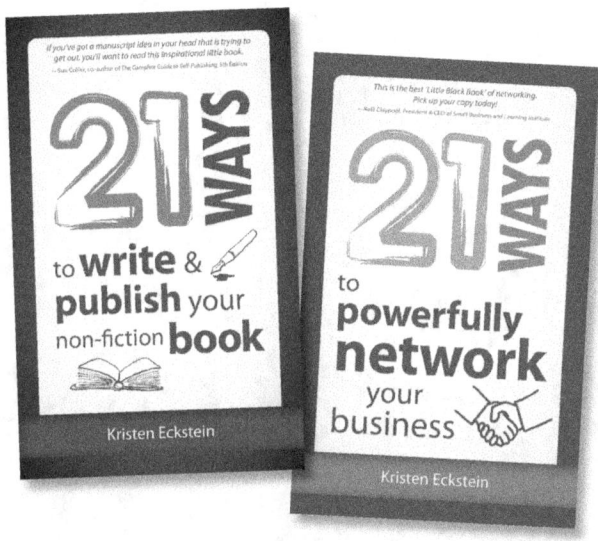

Don't miss a single book in the series!

Look for more *21 Ways*™ books at:

21WaysBooks.com

www.ingramcontent.com/pod-product-compliance
Lightning Source LLC
Chambersburg PA
CBHW052110070526
44584CB00017B/2424